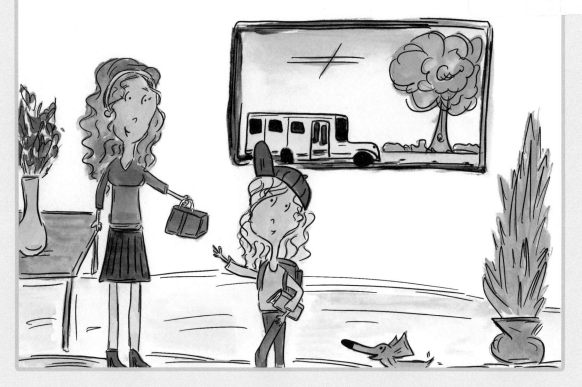

When I woke up, I thought it would be a normal day.
Little did I know that my battle
with one angry worm was about to start.

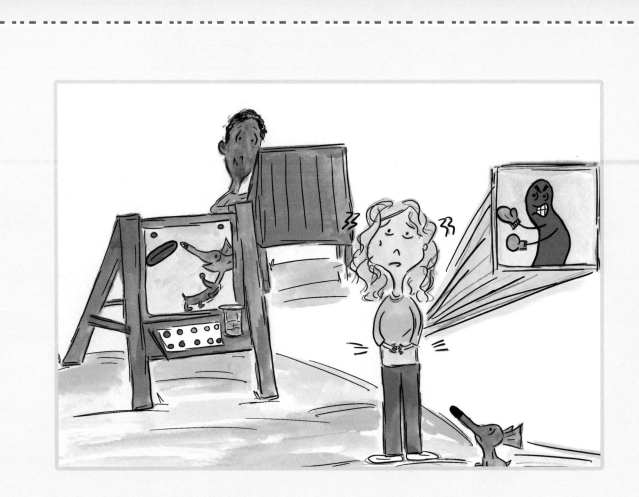

I went to school and had made it halfway through art class when I felt a strange feeling in my stomach, right by my belly button. It felt like someone was poking me, HARD! I almost yelled!

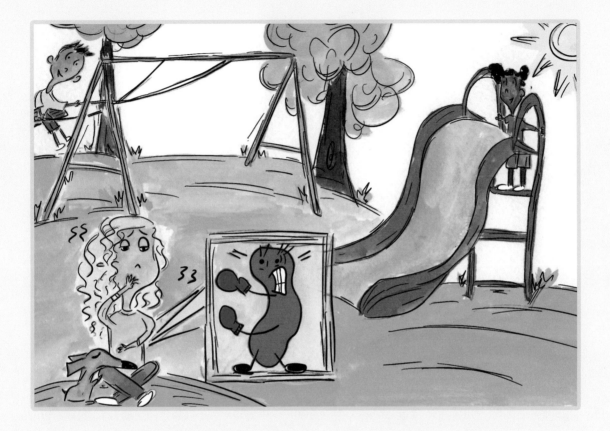

The feeling went away but only for a little.
By recess, it had come back – full force attack.
It felt like someone was punching me from the inside.
Punches at my belly button and then down to my lower
right side. The battle had started!

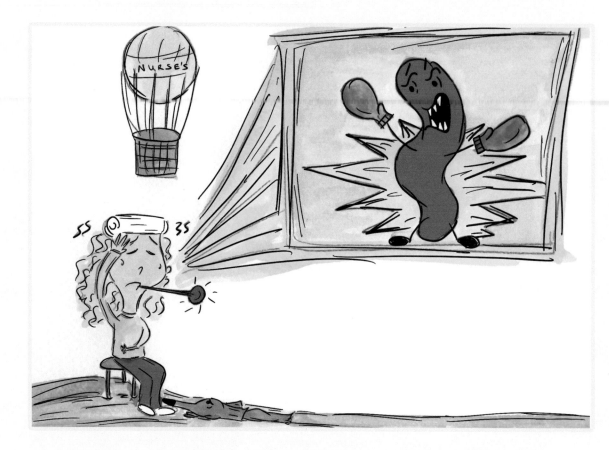

I went to the nurse who said I was running hot like
a steam engine! She tried to get me to eat something but the
punching in my stomach was not making me hungry. My family
arrived and they decided it was time to call in the reinforcements
so we went to the doctor's office.

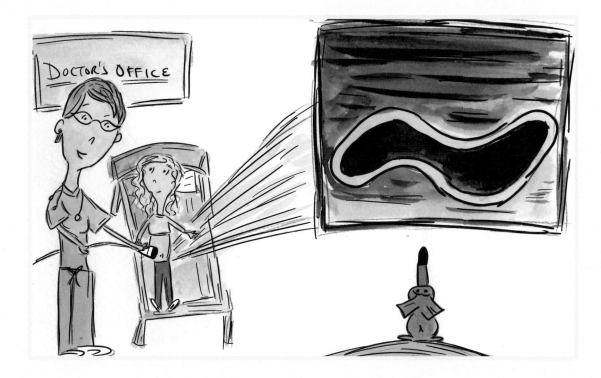

The doctor took a picture of my belly
and said I had **appendicitis**.
Appen-di-what?? Appendicitis.
My family looked concerned. I looked confused.
That's when my surgeon was called.

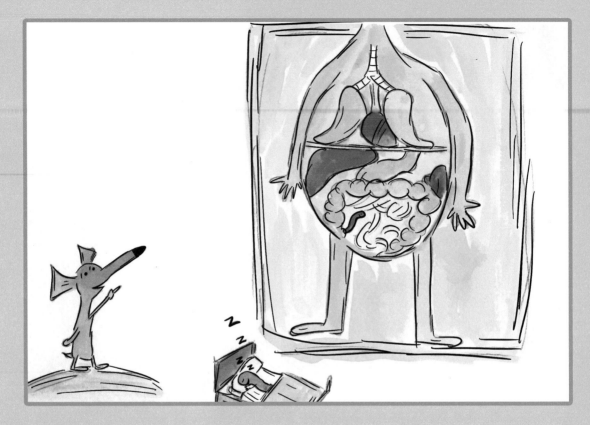

My surgeon said an appendix is a piece of intestine that lives in my belly and is shaped like a big worm. It is attached to the first piece of my large intestine (the **cecum**). It usually lives a very boring life like a cat. It has no job, just lies in my belly, and naps most of the day. But sometimes, something can cause it to get blocked up.

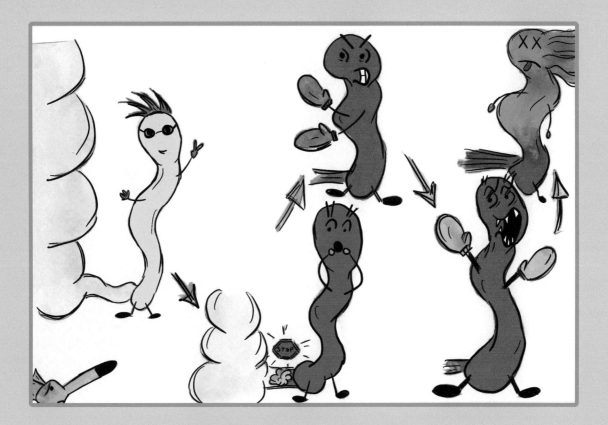

This makes it get big, red, and angry. It goes from a peaceful existence to waging war on my insides. Sometimes it may even explode (called **perforated appendicitis**)! It was time to fight back and get that worm out of my belly!

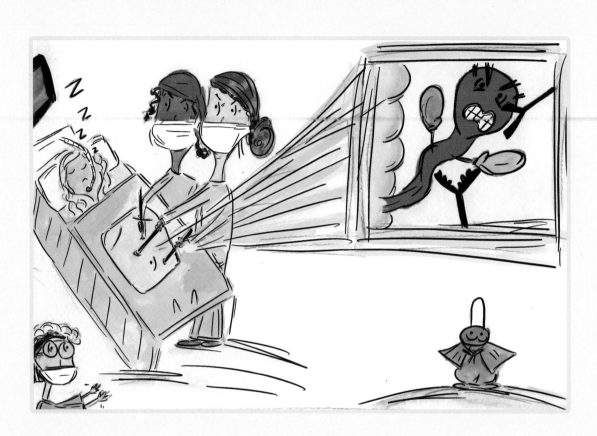

My surgeon took me to the operating room where I fell
asleep. She said I would not feel a single thing; only the
worm would! She made three itty bitty cuts in my belly
and put her tools in. She found the worm and wow,
did it look mad!

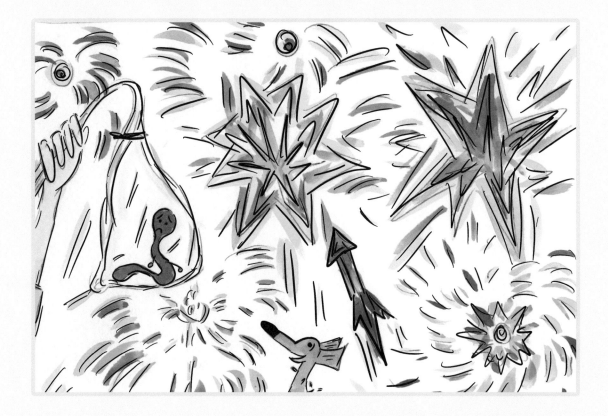

It dodged and tried to hide from the attack. But my surgeon was too quick. She grabbed it and pulled it right out of my belly! The battle had been won! The angry worm was defeated!

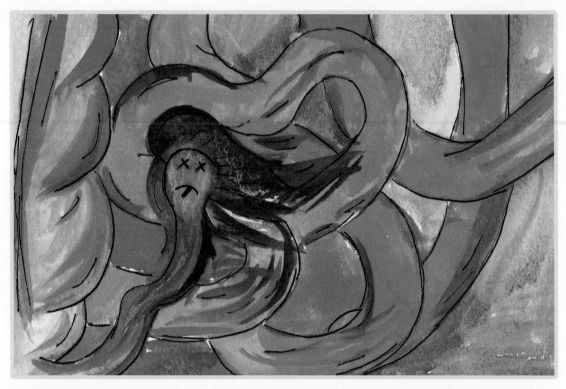

Now, what if the worm had exploded (**perforated**)? When an appendix gets so big, mad, and angry, it can burst into pieces! If your surgeon recommends surgery, they will try to find what is left of the worm and clean up the mess it caused the best they can. Sometimes your surgeon will not recommend surgery and fight the battle instead with special medicines (called **antibiotics**) and possibly a **drain** (a small tube to help clear out the mess).

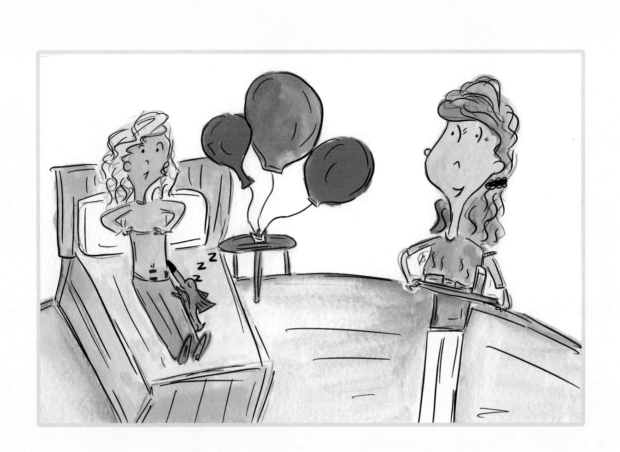

When I woke up after surgery, my belly hurt but in a different way. Now it just felt like I had run around the playground ten times too many. My nurse said I'd start feeling even better tomorrow. And once I was eating, I would be able to go home; usually within the same day!

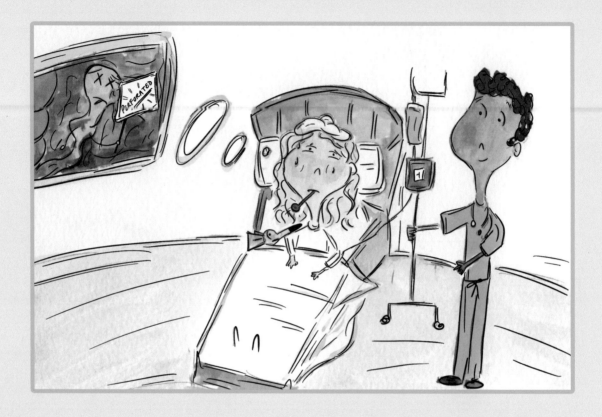

Now if your worm exploded, you will stay in the
hospital longer. Your belly may still hurt a little more and for
a little longer, and you'll be on antibiotics to help fight the
mess the angry worm left behind. Sometimes, you may feel
nauseous and even vomit.

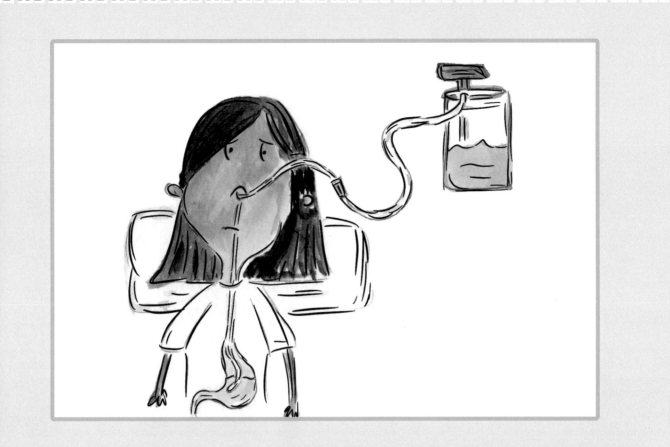

If you do, you may need a special tube put in your nose (called a **nasogastric tube**), which will help you feel better. Soon you'll be able to eat and drink again without feeling sick. You'll even start farting and pooping again (your surgeon will be super happy about that; gosh, doctors are weird!). Then it will be time to go home!

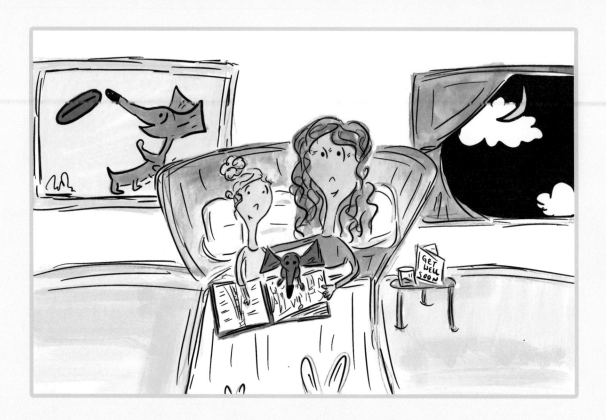

When I got home, I read a story about another kid's battle with an angry worm. Turns out everyone has a worm in their belly but only some of the worms are silly enough to try to wage war. But don't worry. If they do, I know the doctors will be there to fight back!

Facts

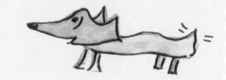

1. Appendicitis is the most common cause of sudden belly pain in kids and teenagers. There are about 70,000 cases in kids every year in the United States.

2. It is caused by a blockage of poop, mucus, or inflamed tissue. This makes the appendix get angry and infected.

3. Appendicitis often happens between the ages of 10 and 19 years old; but really, it can happen at any age!

4. Usually it starts with pain near your belly button (**periumbilical pain**) that moves to your right lower side. You may feel nauseous or vomit, not want to eat, and may have a fever.

5. If you are sick for more than two days, sometimes your appendix can explode (**perforate**), spilling infection into your belly. Usually with perforated appendicitis, you have a higher fever and your belly is extra tender.

6. To diagnose appendicitis, you may have an **ultrasound** that shows a BIG appendix with fluid around it, meaning it's infected.

7. If the ultrasound cannot find the appendix, (which happens a lot), we may get a **CT scan** which is an even better way to see it. Other times, we may just watch you in the hospital overnight and see if you get better or worse because a stomach bug can act like appendicitis.

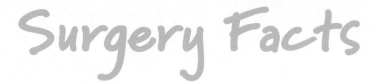

Surgery Facts

1. In non-perforated appendicitis, we usually recommend surgery to remove the appendix (called **Appendectomy**). This is usually done as a **Laparoscopic Appendectomy**, which means with little incisions and a camera. The risks of surgery include infection, bleeding, and damage to surrounding structures. These problems are all very rare.

2. In perforated appendicitis, we may recommend surgery. But if the appendix has been perforated for a while, we may not recommend surgery right away. If we do not perform surgery right away, we will bring you into the hospital for antibiotics. We may also place a **percutaneous drain** in your belly to help clear out the mess. We often plan for surgery about 6 weeks later, called an '**interval appendectomy**.'

3. Do not eat or drink anything for 8 hours before surgery!

4. The surgery incisions will be three tiny cuts in your belly, or just one at your bellybutton, about the size of your fingernail. You will be asleep so you won't feel a thing.

5. When you wake up, you will have small bandages with blue glue or tape underneath them. This glue or tape will peel off on its own in several weeks. Do not peel if off yourself as it helps your cuts heal.

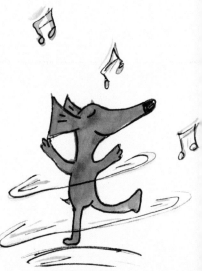

After Surgery

1. You can go home once you are eating and your pain is okay. Usually this is about 4-6 hours after surgery if your appendix was non-perforated.

2. Alternate taking acetaminophen and ibuprofen at home for your pain. Sometimes we may give you a stronger medicine as well, called an opioid. Use the opioid only if your pain is still very bad. Opioids may cause constipation.

3. You can shower right away. Do not soak in a tub or go swimming for 5 days.

4. Don't lift any heavy objects for 2 weeks after surgery. Otherwise your incisions may not heal.

5. Call your doctor for worsening belly pain, fevers higher than 101 °F, vomiting, and/or wounds that become red and leak fluid.

6. You may see your surgeon about 2 weeks after surgery to make sure you are doing well.

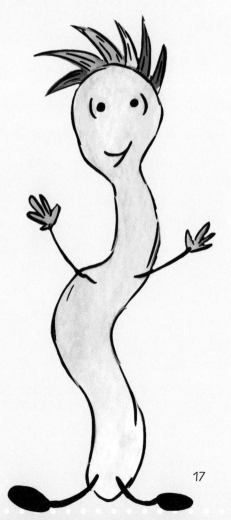

Perforated Appendix

1. You may feel sick for 5-7 days, or more, since your appendix exploded and left quite a mess!

2. You can eat and drink if you feel like it. If you start feeling sick, stop.

3. You may be on antibiotics for 7-14 days to help fight the infection.

4. You may get an '**ileus.**' This means your intestines stop working because of the mess your appendix made. You may feel sick to your stomach and even throw up. Your stomach may also feel extra big like a tight drum.

5. If you have an 'ileus,' you may need a special tube that goes into your nose. It's called a **nasogastric tube** (NG tube for short). It will help you feel better by keeping your stomach empty.

6. Once you start farting and pooping, it means your intestines are working again! This can take a couple of days to a week, or even longer.

7. You can go home once you no longer have a fever, are pooping, are eating, AND you pain is controlled.

8. You are at risk for a belly infection or **abscess**. This happens several weeks later in 10-20% of kids. You will start feeling sick again and have a fever. You will need to come back to the hospital to get more antibiotics and get a small **drain** to clean out the abscess.

9. The drain is placed in your belly while you are asleep and removed after several days.

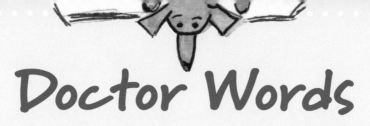

Doctor Words

Infection: An attack from germs in the body, that happens if you have non-perforated or perforated appendicitis. We fight it with antibiotics.

Ultrasound: A safe, painless way to take a picture of your appendix and see if it's sick using high-frequency sound waves without radiation.

CT scan: A painless picture of your body using a small amount of radiation. You lie in a machine shaped like a small tunnel that takes lots of pictures.

Antibiotics: Medicines that help fight appendicitis, by fighting infection. You will get them before surgery and after surgery if your appendix perforated.

Percutaneous drain: This is a small plastic tube that is placed in your belly. It is used to clear out the mess left from a perforated appendix or to drain an abscess.

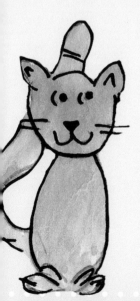

It is placed in your belly by our radiology friends (a special kind of doctor) while you are asleep, so you won't feel a thing.

Ruptured appendicitis: Another name for perforated appendicitis.

Fecalith: A stone made from poop that can block the appendix and cause appendicitis. Not everyone has a fecalith.

Cecum: The first part of your large intestine. This is where your appendix lives!

Meet the Author:
Dr. Maria Baimas-George

Maria Baimas-George MD MPH is a surgeon, training to specialize in abdominal transplantation. Inspired by her patients and mentors, she writes and illustrates books explaining medical and surgical conditions to children and their loved ones. Her goal is to create books that provide useful information to help with understanding and to offer comfort and hope.

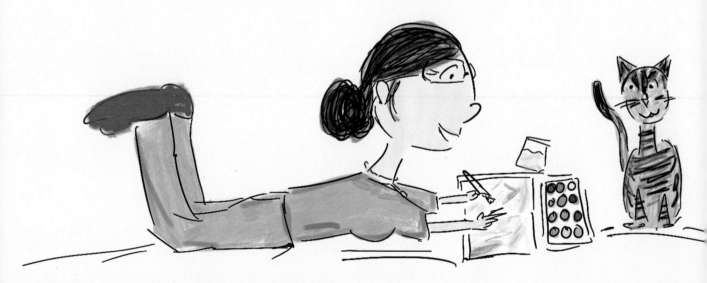